First Ever Book Focused on Safety in MRI Rooms in India

SIMPLIFYING MRI SAFETY

Implementable Strategies for ZERO Accidents

AF657979

First Ever Book Focused on Safety in MRI Rooms in India

SIMPLIFYING MRI SAFETY

Implementable Strategies for ZERO Accidents

Shveta Dang

Worldwide Published by
Pendown Press

PENDOWN PRESS LLP
An ISO 9001 & ISO 14001 Certified Co.,
Regd. Office: 3767A, Kanhaiya Nagar,
Tri Nagar, Delhi-110035
Ph.: 8130886000, 9650072927, 8595249536
E-mail: info@pendownpress.com
Branch Office: 1A/2A, 20, Hari Sadan, Ansari Road,
Daryaganj, New Delhi-110002
Ph.: 011-45794768
Website: PendownPress.com

Edition: 2025
Price: ₹ 399/-
ISBN: 978-93-6338-473-6

All Rights Reserved
All the ideas and thoughts in this book are given by the author and she is responsible for the treatise, facts and dialogues used in this book. She is also responsible for the used pictures and the permission to use them in this book. Copyright of this book is reserved with the author. The publisher does not have any responsibility for the above-mentioned matters. No part of this publication may be reproduced, distributed, or transmitted in any form or by any means, including photocopying, recording, or other electronic or mechanical methods, without the prior written permission of the publisher and author.

Layout and Cover Designed by Pendown Graphics Team
Printed and Bound in India by Thomson Press India Ltd.

Dedicated

to my Father...

Late Shri. Subhash Dang

Table of Contents

CHAPTER 6: **SECRET #6**

CHAPTER 7

CHAPTER 8

Acknowledgements

Just as MRI safety is a collective responsibility, this book represents the culmination of collaboration and contributions from numerous individuals and organizations dedicated to advancing MRI safety in India. I express my deepest gratitude to all who have played a role in shaping this work.

First and foremost, I extend my sincere appreciation to the Radiology healthcare professionals who generously shared their insights, experiences, and case studies. Your dedication on the front lines and your willingness to contribute have been pivotal in shaping the practical dimensions of this book.

I am profoundly grateful to my mentors, Tobias Gilk and Dr. Emanuel Kanal, whose teachings provided me with a comprehensive and in-depth understanding of the subject. Your guidance has been invaluable in my journey toward greater expertise in MRI safety.

A heartfelt thank you to Metrasens for allowing me to reference their studies and use their images. Your commitment to promoting MRI safety through innovative products and data sharing has been instrumental to this endeavor.

I extend my deepest thanks to my family and friends for their constant support and belief throughout the writing process. Special acknowledgment goes to my first coach my mother, Sunila Dang, my life coach, Akshar Yadav, and my partner, Rohan Mehtani. Your unwavering belief in me, even during moments of self-doubt, has been a cornerstone of my perseverance.

Finally, I wish to express my appreciation to the publishing team for their editorial expertise and dedication to bringing this book to life.

To all who endeavor to enhance MRI safety, your efforts serve as an enduring source of inspiration. I hope this book proves to be a valuable resource in promoting patient safety and fostering a culture of continuous improvement.

Disclaimer

The advice and opinions shared in this book are based on the author's personal experience and are intended to raise awareness about MRI safety for both staff and patients. While every effort has been made to provide accurate and practical insights, readers are encouraged to use their discretion and refer to official guidelines, institutional protocols, and expert consultations when implementing any recommendations. The author shall not be held liable for any decisions, actions, or outcomes resulting from the use of the information in this book.

Foreword

This book will change your life!
And yes, that is its intention.

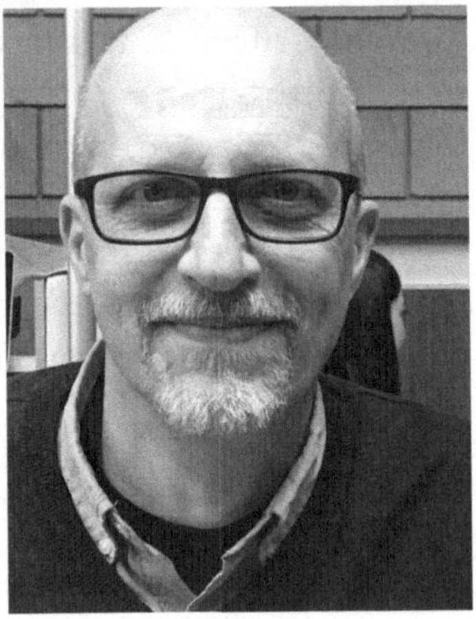

This book is meant to help MRI providers across India from making mistakes that have previously resulted in injury and death. It's meant to allow you to get a good night's sleep, knowing you've taken all the steps to protect patients, radiographers, and staff from preventable MRI accidents.

It's meant to prevent the guilt and shame that might consume you by preventing an accident that could ruin someone's life. This book arms you, the reader, with the knowledge of how your actions can prevent these tragedies.

Shveta Dang, the author, might best be described as India's 'Godmother of MRI Safety,' and she has laid out, in very straightforward and direct terms what many of the greatest MRI risks are, and the steps that MRI providers can take to dramatically reduce them. I hope you take her guidance to heart and make sure that your MRI service is built around MRI safety's best practices.

Tobias Gilk

International MRI Safety Trainer.

Endorsement

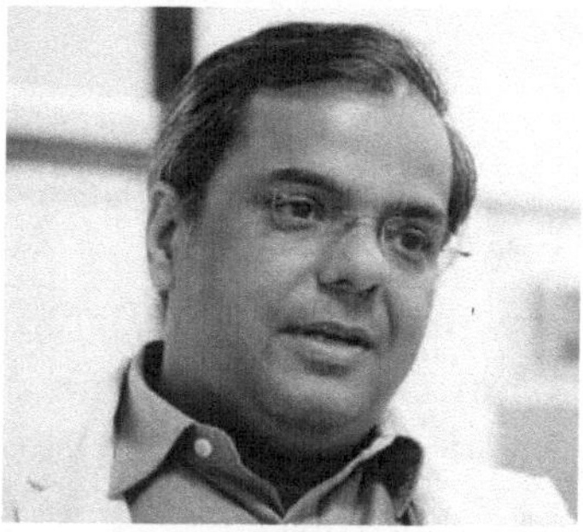

I've known Shveta for the last five years as a passionate proponent of MR safety. Her passion in this field is infectious and extremely motivational to the radiology fraternity, where MRI imaging plays a critical and large role. Her willingness to educate and upskill all levels of MR personnel is truly a rare trait and exemplifies her passion for this very critical aspect of medicine – **"Do no Harm"**

She is always a call away to support our staff in times of need. She has generously shared her extensive experience in Indian MRI rooms, providing our teams with regular training on the critical nuances of MRI safety. Her willingness to provide training and retraining ensures that all MR personnel are upskilled and updated regularly through this re-enforcement. Her guidance has been instrumental in reviewing and strengthening our safety systems and protocols.

Through her unwavering support and expertise, she has played a pivotal role in enhancing our knowledge, bringing us closer to our goal of achieving zero accidents in the MRI environment and keeping patients safe.

Dr. Bharat Aggarwal

Principal Director, Radiology Services,
Max Healthcare

Meet your secret teller & discover what makes her so passionate about MRI safety

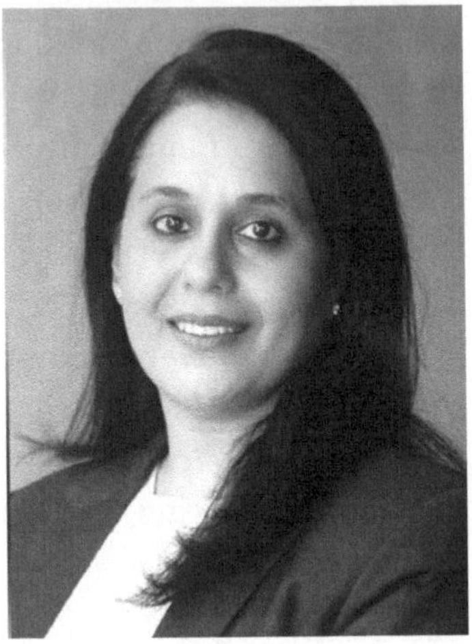

Hello, Thank you for choosing this book.

My name is Shveta Dang, and **I am the first Indian MRI Safety Trainer.**

I had the privilege of training under the expert guidance of global MRI safety trainers, some of whom were members of the ACR 2012 and 2016 committees.

My journey with MRI began ten years ago at the start of my career with Marrsis Disha, pioneers in introducing MRI-conditional products in India. Today, they hold the largest portfolio of MRI-conditional products in the country, dedicated to advancing MRI safety. During my time with Marrsis Disha, I gained hands-on experience and expertise in installing MRI-conditional products and ensuring the safety of patients and equipment in MRI facilities across the nation. I also collaborated with prominent health agencies in India, such as HLL, to raise awareness about MRI safety and identify equipment suitable for MRI environments. Many of these initiatives have been successfully implemented in new hospitals.

In 2018, a personal incident solidified my passion for MRI safety. It was a regular visit to a hospital MRI with a radiologist. However, he had accidentally forgotten a sharp object in his pocket. As soon as we entered the MRI gantry room the object was drawn across the room by the MRI's magnetic field, narrowly missing me and striking the machine.

The incident was not only alarming but also revealing—the radiologist remained unaware of the severity of the situation. This was a turning point for me, emphasizing the critical need for MRI safety awareness in India.

When I further discovered that there was a lack of resources available in India focusing on MRI Safety education it further inspired me to pursue formal training outside India, bring the education back to our country, and dedicate myself to educating others about this overlooked but vital area.

Since 2021, I have trained approximately 4,500 professionals from renowned institutions like AIIMS, PGI, Tata Memorial, Tata Trust, Max Group, and Fortis Group. My efforts have focused on promoting MRI safety and fostering safe practices in their hospitals.

The journey so far has been brilliant.

So why this book?

You must be wondering why I am sharing this free book when I can charge a premium for sharing this information.

After all, if you implement the concepts shared in this book you can actually move towards creating a safer MRI Environment in your hospital. Besides you must be wary because we all are often taught that there are no free lunches in life. Well, rest assured, there is no hidden agenda here.

As someone deeply passionate about MRI safety, it pains me to hear so many myths circulating in the industry without addressing the real issues.

- **These unsubstantiated myths have unfortunately made achieving our safety goals seem unattainable. I am committed to debunking these myths and shifting the spotlight onto MRI safety, highlighting the pertinent issues and their practical solutions, What better than sharing them as a book— a ready reference for whenever needed?**
- **Furthermore, I recognize that I cannot personally coach everyone, which is why I aim to share my expertise on MRI safety with as many people as possible. I want to empower a wide audience with practical knowledge on implementing basic measures for safer MRIs. So of course a book to reach the maximum number of people without time and logistic constraints.**

I am confident that the subjects addressed in this book will demonstrate how practical and critical it is to implement MRI safety measures, making it accessible and understandable for everyone. Together, let's commit to ensuring that MRIs are safe environments for all.

If you encounter any challenges, we are here to support you throughout your journey.

Yours,

Shveta Dang,

MRI Safety Enthusiast

SECRET - 1

THE BIG SECRET NOBODY TELLS YOU

MRI MAY NOT BE THE "SAFEST" DIAGNOSTIC MODALITY

MAGNETIC PROBLEM ACCIDENTS ARE INCREASING 4 FOLDS

MRI Scans are on the increase and along with the same there is an increase in the strength of the MRI Magnets.

There is a constant battle between the manufacturing companies about the magnetic field strength which has increased from 0.35 Tesla earlier to 7 Tesla magnets in our lifetimes and now the world is talking about 11 Tesla and higher magnets. Who knows how powerful the magnets will be in the future?

This increase in the strength of the MRI magnet provides better information for the radiologist and he can infer and diagnose better from the detailed scans.

While the MRI modality itself is safe the increase in magnetic strength does bring its own challenges from an MRI safety perspective.

A 3 T MRI scanner is around 60,000 times stronger than the Earth's magnetic field. And this strong magnetic field requires special attention.

While there are exhaustive trainings conducted about how to use the functions in these new MRIs, rarely ever is there any discussion on what to avoid when being in the MRI environment or what to do to avoid accidents in the MRI Room.

There is lesser awareness of the basic Dos and Dont's in an MRI environment to keep the patient, equipment, and staff safe. This adds to the risk and leads to accidents. As per studies conducted globally, it has been proven that with the increase in the number of MRI scans MRI accidents have also increased fourfold.

Given the high magnetic strength, the accidents in the MRI are in no way minor and there is a huge chance of fatality, big injuries, or damage to the equipment.

All the above factors are a reason good enough to focus on MRI safety as an important aspect.

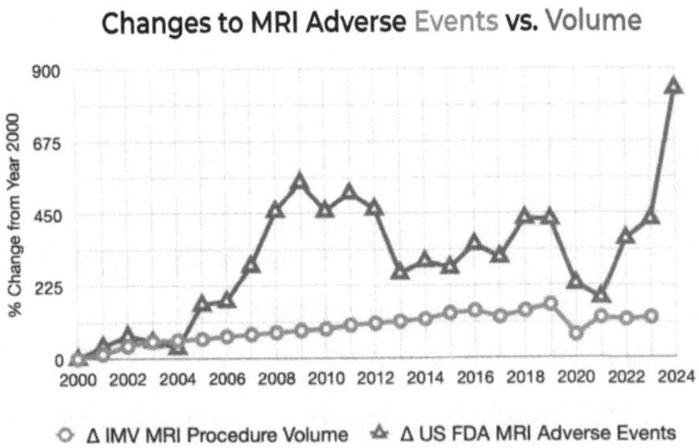

Image Courtesy: Gilk Radiology Consultant.com

If we talk about India in particular, as per a study in 2020 there was 1 machine per 10 million people in India as opposed to 1 machine per 1.5 million people in most developed nations.

This puts a huge load on the current MRI setup in our country. The consultants and radiologists are doing a great job in handling the workload. However, the huge load of the number of patients being scanned every day and the lack of focus on MRI Safety education in India aggravates the issues involved.

Another point to ponder over from the safety angle is that the MRI facility is used not only by radiologists but also by multiple other disciplines like Anaesthesia or Critical Care where a lot of OT staff accompany their patients under anaesthesia to the MRI room as these patients need to be monitored constantly. Most of this staff who are very well versed with their subject and area of expertise are not aware of how the MRI room is different from their OT room and the implications and hazards of the strong magnetic field.

Given the gravity of the accidents that can happen in the MRI environment, it is imperative that the multi-disciplinary staff members also be made aware of the dos and don'ts as well, when on the MRI premises.

Many of the reported and non-reported accidents happen in off hours when the hospitals are most minimally staffed and this adds a certain level of complexity to the situation.

Accidents Don't Care For The Time Of The Day

India 2014: One of the First Reported Accidents

Take for example the big accident at a hospital in the Western part of the country where a person was stuck to the MRI bore for 7 hours which led to permanent injuries. This took place late in the evening when most of the day staff and heads had already left for the day.

India 2023: The Case of The Misjudged Cleaning Equipment

A similar incident happened at a hospital in the East. During the off hours, a new cleaning staff member who was unaware of how the MRI room is different from other rooms in the hospital and believed that the huge machine would be "off" just like other equipment in the hospital are in off hours, ended up carrying ferrous cleaning material into the MRI environment. The cleaning material flew like a projectile and stuck to the magnet. Thankfully no one got injured here.

There are many many more similar examples to quote happening regularly in every part of the country. All these do bring attention to the fact that given the MRI Accidents can happen at any time, the MRI processes and facilities need to be planned in such a way that there should be restricted access to the MRI gantry room and any resource who can access these premises needs to be trained and be fully aware of the potential hazards in and around the strong magnetic strengths.

That said, MRI accidents have also happened during the daytime which has led to the loss of life, and property, a lot of financial losses and in most cases the loss of the reputation of the hospital.

Most of the MRI accidents are not documented as there is no mandate to document the same and also unfortunately sometimes especially for burn and auditory damages people are unaware of what happened as the symptoms appear a day or two later.

The issue that stems here is that it is difficult for hospitals to believe that MRI Accidents are such a big problem. However, having interacted with multiple hospitals across India, I can tell you with certainty that MRI Accidents whether documented or not, happen everywhere.

So we need to be on guard as to how we can avoid these accidents.

- But what is it exactly that we are looking to guard for?
- What causes these accidents?
- Are they even avoidable?
- And who needs to be focusing on avoiding these accidents?
- End of the day who's responsible for MRI Safety?

The list of these questions in your mind right now would be endless.

Through the next chapters, you will get the answers to most of these questions.

So let us get started.

SECRET - 2

THE MAGNETIC KILLER CAN BE A THREAT TO LIVES AND REPUTATION

The inherent high magnetic field strength of clinical MR imaging units poses a risk for projectile injury to personnel in the MRI environment or MR imaging equipment damage.

Let's get the basics straight first:
What is a projectile and how does it happen?

The static magnetic field of an MRI scanner exerts forces on ferromagnetic and other magnetic materials in its vicinity. These forces can draw unrestrained objects, making them airborne, towards and into the scanner's magnet bore with very high speed and force. This phenomenon is known as the projectile effect and can result in catastrophic consequences for individuals in the path of the projectile and significant damage to equipment. To avoid serious or fatal injury from projectiles, MR personnel must understand the principles of the projectile effect and properly screen individuals before entering the scanner room for ferromagnetic objects.

Even in the absence of patient harm, the financial consequences of interrupted patient throughput or

equipment damage, including emergency shutdown of the MRI scanner, resulting from ferromagnetic projectiles can be significant.

The first reported MRI Projectile Accident took place in 2001 in the US. A 6-year-old boy succumbed to his injuries when a ferromagnetic oxygen tank mistakenly made it to the MRI examination room becoming a projectile, then flew through the air at 20 to 30 feet per second, and fractured the boy's skull.

And ever since there have been multiple such cases reported worldwide. Let's look at a few accidents reported globally and in India.

INDIA 2018: The Case of the Misjudged Oxygen Cylinder

Back in 2018, in a busy hospital, a lady was called in for an MRI Scan. For some reason, someone called for oxygen for the lady. An ignorant attendant hurriedly rushed inside the MRI carrying a ferrous Oxygen cylinder. He was immediately pulled in along with the Oxygen cylinder which opened and the force of the oxygen ruptured his lungs causing immediate death. The lady who had come for the scan also suffered injuries.

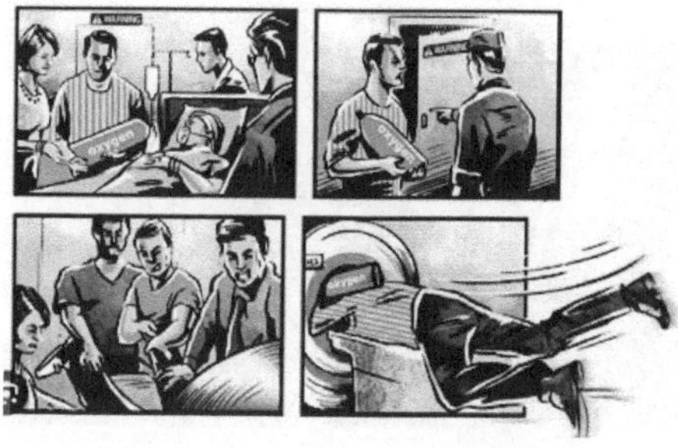

Image Courtesy: https://www.dnaindia.com/mumbai/report-mumbai-mri-death-case-freak-mishap-turns-into-blame-game-2579317

USA 2023: The Case of Security Lax: Relying on the Patient's Word

In an unusual incident recently, a woman in the United States was shot in her right buttock area after she took a loaded gun into an MRI machine during a doctor's visit back in June 2023.

According to the US Food and Drug Administration, the 57-year-old, had a handgun concealed on her person as she was slid into the MRI machine. When being verbally questioned before the scan if she was carrying any ferrous material, the lady denied it. However, when the machine's powerful magnets were engaged, the metal trigger of the handgun tripped and the firearm discharged causing her injury.

INDIA 2020: The Case of the Ambulance Driver

An ambulance driver who was " trying to help" a patient unknowing of the MRI scanner's magnetic strength carried a ferrous oxygen cylinder and got stuck in the MRI machine. He claimed he was sucked in and managed to free his stuck palm.

Fortunately, the 40-year-old escaped with a fractured little finger on the righthand.

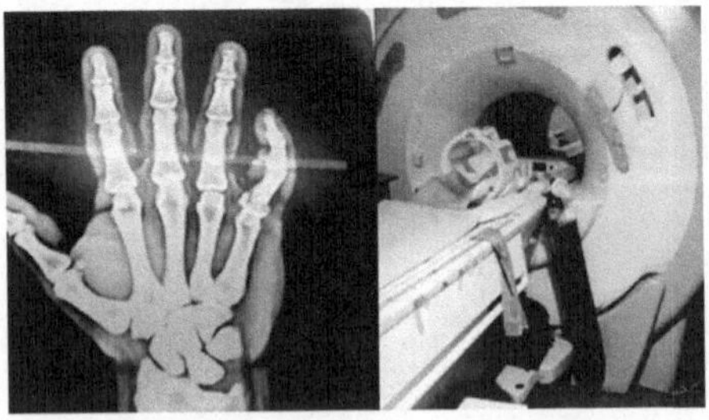

Image courtesy:https://www.mid-day.com/mumbai/mumbai-news/article mumbai-man-sucked-in-by-mri-machine-gets-away-with-just-a-broken-finger-23183247\

The list of projectile accidents is endless. Such incidents underscore the critical need for thorough screening and safety checks to ensure that no ferromagnetic objects are brought into the MRI room.

How do we ensure that no potentially hazardous ferromagnetic objects are brought into the MRI facilities? Are there any more points of caution?

Is there a framework to avoid such accidents?

Read on to know...

SECRET - 3

69% OF MRI PROJECTILE ACCIDENTS CAN BE AVOIDED WITH JUST THESE 3 STEPS

The MRI projectile hazard is a most significant concern in MRI safety, referring to the risk of ferromagnetic objects being attracted to the strong magnetic field of the MRI machine and becoming dangerous projectiles. These projectiles can pose serious life risks to patients, staff, and anyone else in the vicinity of the MRI room They have also damaged the MRI Scanner equipment hence leading to huge financial losses.

As per a study done by Metrasens on reported MRI accidents, it is possible to reduce MRI projectile Accidents by 69% by following three simple steps.

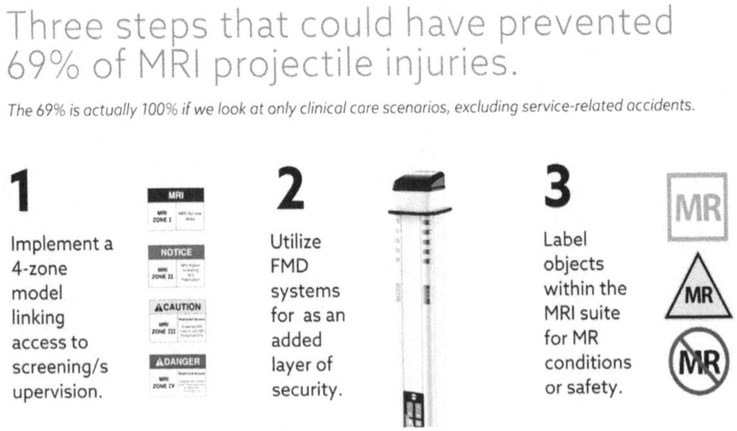

Image Courtesy: Metrasens, UK.

A 69% reduction in MRI projectile accidents is a great number to begin with.

I am sure you would be wondering: What would it take to achieve the same?

Well just like Metrasens, UK explained it's just 3 simple steps that need to be followed.

Let's look at the three steps that can help you achieve this goal.

Step 1: Implementing a 4-Zone Strategy

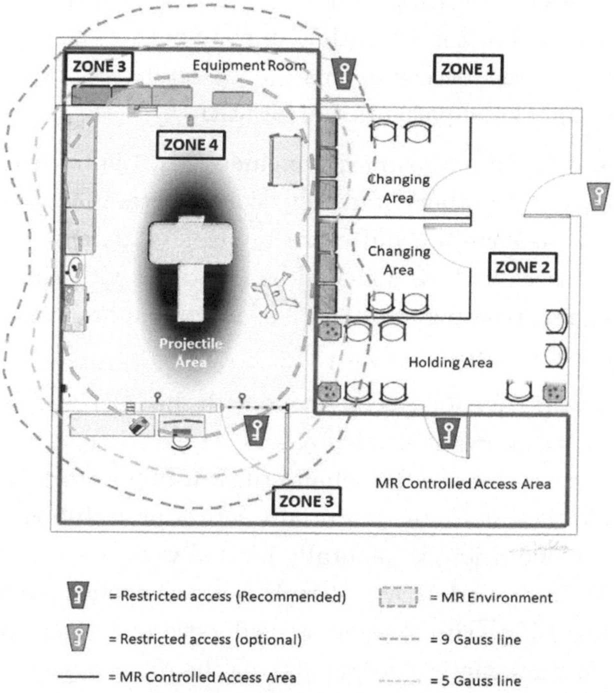

Image Courtesy: ACR 2024 guidelines Chapter 3 MRI Safety Zones

The American College of Radiology has defined four safety Zones within MRI facilities, numbered 1- 4. The Zones correspond to the increasing exposure to the magnetic field, and, therefore, the increasing potential safety risks.

- **Zone 1:** This region includes all areas that are freely accessible to the general public. This area is outside the MR facility itself and is the area through which patients, health care personnel, and other employees of the MR facility access the MR environment.
- **Zone 2:** This area is the interface between the publicly accessible, uncontrolled Zone 1 and the strictly controlled areas of Zones 3 and 4. This area typically contains a patient waiting area, patient preparation areas, locker rooms, etc. Screening and ferromagnetic detection are often performed in Zone 2. Although not a part of the Controlled Access Area, access to this area is often restricted to MR Personnel and patients due for MRI.
- **Zone 3:** Zone 3 primarily includes MR Controlled Access Areas where there is direct doorway access to Zone 4. A common Zone 3 could serve multiple scanners (Zone 4s). Entrances to Zone 3 should be identified with appropriate signage denoting the Zone 3 space and appropriate access control utilized.
- **Zone 4:** Zone 4 is synonymous with the MRI scanner room and is comprised of the physical walled confines where the scanner is located. It includes the MR Projectile Area where there is a definite, potentially lethal projectile risk. Zone 4, by definition, is generally located within a surrounding MR Controlled Access Area. Strictly controlled entrance to Zone 4 is a critical safety consideration for the prevention of ferromagnetic objects entering the room.

SHVETA'S PRO SAFETY TIP

The intent should be to create a ferrous-free Zone 4 and a minimal ferrous Zone 3.

Step 2: Identify all equipment and furniture in the MRI Suite and Label these on the ACR-based MR Labeling guidelines

The MRI scanner room and the surrounding Zones can have multiple equipment/furniture. What needs attention is the ones entering Zone 3 and definitely Zone 4.

The three major categories of products in these Zones are:

- Patient support equipment like monitors, anaesthesia workstations, injectors, etc.
- Furniture for patient transportation like wheelchairs, trolleys, etc.
- On-patient devices which include implants inside the body as well as the devices on the patient's body like CGMs, insulin patches, etc

All these category objects entering Zone 4 need to be classified and labelled.

The ACR guidelines classify three categories for labelling any MRI products:

- MR Safe
- MR Unsafe
- MR Conditional

MRI Labels

Image Courtesy: ACR 2024 Guidelines Chapter 10: CHAPTER 10: Classification of Objects and Medical Implants and Devices in The MR Environment: FDA labelling criteria developed by ASTM International for objects and devices taken into Zone IV [1,2].

The square green MR Safe label is for nonmetallic, nonconducting objects; the triangular yellow label is for objects with MR Conditional labelling; and the round red label is for MR Unsafe objects. Alternatively, these symbols may be printed as black-and-white icons.

As per the ACR guidelines

- **MR Safe:** A designation indicating that the object or device is safe in all MR environments, without conditions. The term "MR Safe" is reserved for items that are composed of materials that are nonmetallic, nonconducting, and nonmagnetic; such objects pose no known hazards during or resulting from exposure to any MR environment
- **MR Conditional:** A designation indicating that the object or device has been demonstrated to be safely used within the MR environment, provided the specified conditions for safe use (as provided by the manufacturer) are met.
- **MR Unsafe:** An item that poses unacceptable risks to the patient, medical staff, or other persons within the MR environment. These objects cannot/should not be used in the MRI Environment, especially inside the 5 Gauss line.

Shveta's Pro Safety Tip

As a thumb rule: anything that has no label should be considered unsafe till you can determine its nature.

"Assuming" basis no knowledge or "assuming" basis past knowledge can not only be dangerous but can even be fatal when it comes to the MRI environment."

Step 3: Implement A Ferromagnetic Screening System For Patients

A well-designed and implementable screening plan for the personnel entering Zone 3 and Zone 4 is a must to ensure MR safety.

A well-framed screening form is the first and most essential step in this. The screening form should be thoroughly filled out. All sections should be carefully explained to the patient/ guardian. No empty responses should be accepted, and each question must be answered with a yes or no, or specific further information must be provided as requested. It would be helpful if the patient could be informed about the importance of the form being filled out thoroughly and seriously when they fill out the form.

Shveta's Pro Safety Tip

A sample screening form as recommended by the ACR guidelines has been provided at the end.

It would be recommended to customise the same, basis your hospital workflow. Also, the MRI personnel who will access MRI Zone 4 should be screened during their onboarding to identify any potential devices or medical conditions that could impact their or others' safety in the MR environment.

The second important step is the use of a Ferromagnetic Detector System (FMDS) before the patient enters the magnet room to prevent ferrous material from entering and becoming a projectile threat. These systems are designed to detect the smallest of ferrous materials and prevent accidents. The ACR guidelines recommend an always-on system that detects approaching hazards to be able to provide prior warning and help take timely action.

In cases where the patient is unaware of their medical history of implants or in rare cases when they do not reveal either accidentally or deliberately about the ferrous material in/on their body, there needs to be another level of security provided.

Hence screening for ferromagnetic materials by direct inspection and use of a ferromagnetic detection system (FMDS) is recommended prior to entering Zone 3 and Zone 4. Implanted and on-planted medical devices, both MR Conditional and MR Unsafe, may include ferromagnetic material (including batteries) that can lead to FMDS activation and provide a warning to remove the same before it enters Zone 4.

The use of conventional metal detectors that do not specifically differentiate between ferromagnetic and nonferromagnetic materials is not recommended. Also, these are often ignored because of the false alarm causing alarm fatigue.

The use of an FMDS is recommended as an adjunct and not a replacement for thorough and conscientious screening of persons prior to being permitted into Zone 4. FMDS screening helps detect ferromagnetic objects and some medical implants missed during the standard screening.

Shveta's Pro Safety Tip

In addition to the patient, the accompanying attendant if any who will enter Zone 4 should also be screened.Choose an FMDS system that should always be on, provides no break-in detection, and should detect approaching hazards as per the ACR guidelines.

SECRET - 4

MEDICAL IMPLANTS AND DEVICES IN AND ON PATIENTS

A CAUSE OF SERIOUS CONCERN

Electronic devices or ferrous devices implanted inside or on the patient undergoing an MRI Scan are increasing by the day. These devices can interact in several ways with the various magnetic fields potentially leading to adverse events. A study was conducted to find the number of implanted devices in patients. The yearly number of MRI examinations performed in patients with AIMDs, including MR-conditional cardiac devices, MR-nonconditional cardiac devices, and MR-conditional noncardiac devices from 2014 to 2022 at Mayo Clinic Arizona is shown below.

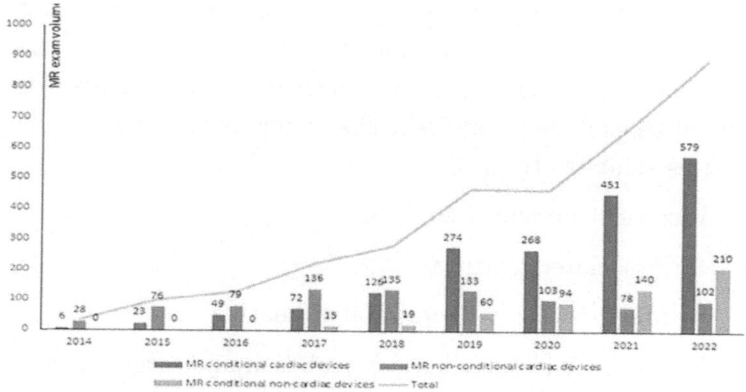

Image Courtesy: https://pubs.rsna.org/doi/abs/10.1148/rg.230102?journalCode=radiographics

The devices can be categorized as active or passive devices.

The most **common types of active implants** are cardiac implantable electronic devices (CIEDs), spinal cord stimulators, deep brain stimulators, bone growth or fusion stimulators, other neurostimulators, and drug infusion pumps.

As more patients with AIMDs undergo MRI, it is important to consider the safety of patients who have these implanted devices during MRI. They can pose dangers as detailed below that in most cases can be fatal. If the implant is not MRI Conditional, the strong magnetic fields can cause:

- Malfunction of the implanted devices
- Displacement of the implanted device
- Temporary or permanent modification of the function
- Inappropriate sensing or triggering of the device

Common passive implants and devices include aneurysm clips, intravascular stents (vascular, ureteral, tracheal, esophageal, etc.), heart valve prostheses, orthopedic implants (plates, screws, pins, total hip prostheses, mesh, etc.), intraocular lens implants and glaucoma shunts, programmable and nonprogrammable ventricular shunts, and prostheses. While they do not have any electronic components, they cannot be excluded from risk. The major risks in MRI of these devices relate to the potential for :

- Electrical current induction,
- RF-associated heating,
- Gradient-associated vibration or heating,
- Magnetic field–associated translation and torque, possible Lenz-related forces.

Let us examine a few real-life scenarios.

United Kingdom 2004:
The Fatal Case of The Missed Pacemaker

In April 2004, a former Mayor in the UK died within minutes of her MRI Scan as her pacemaker malfunctioned under the magnetic effect of the MRI. On investigation, it was found that the screening form was filled purely out of memory and the details of the pacemaker skipped the mind of the attending doctor who referred her to an MRI without checking if the pacemaker was conditional or not.

Pacemaker death after error in hospital

By Paul Stokes

03 April 2004 • 12:01am

A former mayor died after hospital staff failed to note that she had a pacemaker when they sent her for a magnetic scan, an inquest was told.

Molly Brown, 83, was admitted to North Tyneside General Hospital twice within weeks because of blackouts and problems in walking.

Her medical notes made clear reference to the pacemaker, the hearing in Newcastle was told, but the matter "slipped the mind" of a consultant and her notes were not checked by a senior house officer, or read by another house officer or ward sister, when she was sent for an MRI scan.

Mrs Brown, a widow, former borough mayor and magistrate, died as radiowaves from the scan scrambled her pacemaker's settings and interfered with her heart rhythm. Recording a verdict of misadventure, David Mitford, the Newcastle Coroner, said the warning system to prevent such happenings was inadequate.

Image Courtesy: News article - https://www.telegraph.co.uk/news/uknews/1458421/Pacemaker-death-after-error-in-hospital.html

Morphine Malfunction:
The Case of The False Trigger

In another avoidable accident the morphine pump which the patient had been using for four years due to her back pain issues malfunctioned in the MRI. This caused an additional dose of morphine to be delivered which led to the death of the patient.

A woman dies after a resonance 'blows' her morphine pump

The patient had the device for the administration of this opiate four years before because of her back pains

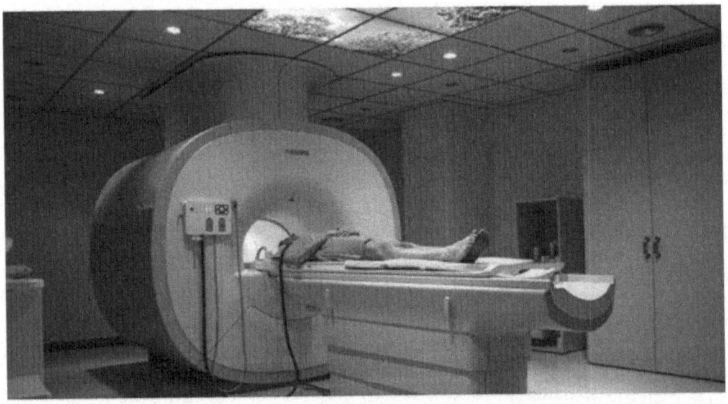

Image Courtesy: https://x.com/tobiasgilk/status/1590343462536155136?mx=2

The 'GOOD NEWS': MRI Implant Hazards Can be Avoided.

While the projectile hazard is easier to identify and counter, the implant hazard requires a lot more careful screening and precaution to be taken. That said this hazard can still be avoided and prevented.

A few steps that could help avoid such accidents

1. The **'Screening Checklist'** should be followed, and the patient should be cross-checked thoroughly for the implants, making sure to make them aware of the consequences of misinformation.
2. Medical records should be cross-checked whenever available to ensure that the information provided by the patient/attendant is correct.
3. Please check and read implant labels carefully to determine their conditionality.
4. FMDS devices can be used in your workflow to detect the minutest of ferrous implants and smaller objects in or on the patient.

> **SHVETA'S PRO SAFETY TIP**
>
> Ensure that the implant labeling is checked and read correctly. An implant that is conditional at 3T MRI might not be conditional at 1.5T MRI.
>
> "Assuming" or "it worked fine when the last MRI was done logic" could cause a significant risk in MRI.

SECRET - 5

THIS UN-NOTICED HAZARD IS A BURNING ISSUE!

Have you ever heard about MRI Burns?

While so many patients undergoing scans in the MRI have experienced these, they are the least documented of all the MRI hazards with the biggest consequences when we look at patient injury.

The time-varying Radiofrequency field which is present only during the MRI Scan is responsible for risks caused by the heating of materials, including human tissues, in the bore of the scanner.

The phenomenon which causes these burns is in most cases one of the below:

1. **Inductive Heating:** The changing magnetic fields generate electrical current which can flow through conductive material i.e. human body in this case. When the electrical current is chanelled into a small area heat is generated which could result in burns.
2. **Proximity Burns:** Burns due to proximity to the scanner walls.
3. **Antenna Effect:** Elongated conductive wires whose length is one-half of the RF wavelength can act as antennas producing currents that are concentrated on the tips causing heat generation.

4. **Another reason for MRI burns could be wearable threats like clothes** that carry invisible metallic fiber. These being superconductors of electricity lead to burns.

We need to pay more attention when sedated patients or paediatrics undergo MRI Scans. Given they are sedated, it is normally too late till the time anyone knows that the burn has happened due to any of the above factors.

Another smaller but known reason is Tattoo Ink Burns. Sometimes there are metal particles present in the Tattoo Ink. The strong magnetic waves push and pull these particles which irritate the skin and in extreme cases may cause burns.

Shveta's Pro Safety Tip

In most cases, the patient does not know that they have suffered burns and only notices the redness post-scan. It turns into a blister or painful burn in the next 12-24 hours which could worsen even more with time depending on the degree of the burn.

This is due to the fact that the burn has happened at a subdermal level and symptoms show up much later.

1°, 2° and 3° burns have occurred in the past in patients undergoing MRI

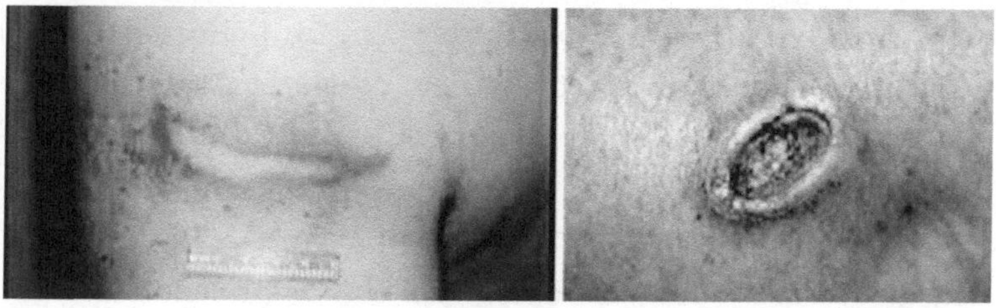

Image courtesy Dr. Joel Femlee, Mayo Clinic
http://www.nationalacademies.org/hmd/~/media/Files/Report%20Files/1999/To-Err-is-Human/To%20Err%20is%20Human%201999%20%20report%20brief.pdf

While in most cases these burns seem unimaginable, there have been cases to prove they can lead to serious injuries. Let's review a few ...

India: The Case of the Sari Catastrophe

A lady in the southern part of India sustained major burns when she got her scan done wearing a sari. The sari was made in the traditional way using gold thread. Gold being a superconductor of current generated heat during the scan causing serious burns.

USA: The Case of Only Burns: No Silver Lining on These Yoga Pants

In another similar incident, one of the latest health clothing brands introduced new Yoga Pants. A patient who was scanned wearing these Yoga pants suffered burns. On analysis, it was found that the Yoga Pants were made with microfibers which were a superconductor leading to generating heat and subsequent burns.

Australia 2024: The Case of Mysterious 2nd° Burns

According to local news coverage, a young toddler girl who went for a normal MRI scan suffered a second-degree burn on her leg. This was discovered when the toddler woke up from sedation and began screaming. Confused and frustrated, the parents took their daughter to a second hospital, where she was diagnosed with a contact burn from an MRI.

The above are a few examples and the list is endless. Just like projectile accidents, there are many incidents reported for MRI-related burns making it a cause of worry and a subject to be paid attention to.

THE GOOD NEWS: 94% of the MRI Burn Accidents can be avoided by following these three simple steps.

As gruesome as the burn injuries seem, almost all of them can be avoided by following best practices

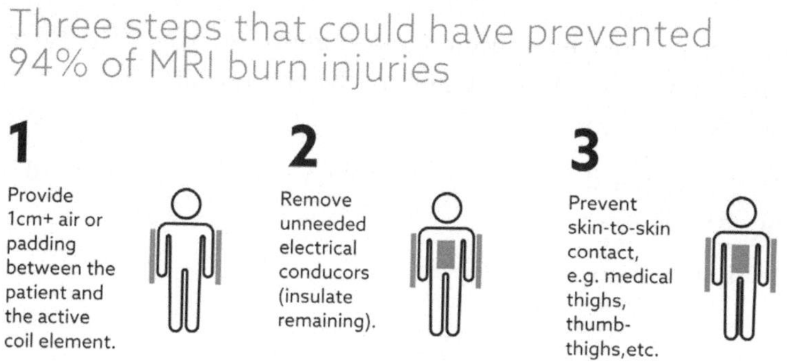
Three steps that could have prevented 94% of MRI burn injuries
1
Provide 1cm+ air or padding between the patient and the active coil element.
2
Remove unneeded electrical conducors (insulate remaining).
3
Prevent skin-to-skin contact, e.g. medical thighs, thumb-thighs,etc.

Image Courtesy: Metrasens, UK.

1. Padding should be provided to patients to ensure body parts do not touch each other.
2. Padding should be provided to patients to ensure their bare body parts do not touch the MRI Bore. The paddings are always supplied by the OEM suppliers along with the MRI scanner.
3. All electrical cables from MRI equipment should be routed out of the MRI in a linear fashion to prevent forming any loops.
4. Ensure the electrical cables are well insulated and they should not touch the bare body of the patient.
5. Patients should also not form loops with their body parts touching each other.
6. Only MRI conditional Carbon electrodes should be used for ECG.
7. Patients should be changed into hospital-provided pocket-free gowns for the scans.

8. Only labelled MRI Conditional accessories should be used inside the MRI room. Any product that does not have a label should be considered unsafe and analyzed accordingly and thoroughly till its nature can be detected before being used in MRI.

Most of the solutions recommended above to avoid MRI Burns can be immediately implemented by the hospital at no extra cost. So why wait?

Have you heard about the "unspoken and unheard hazard in the MRI Room" ...

Read on to know more.

SECRET - 6

"AUDITORY DAMAGE" THE UNHEARD HAZARD OF THE MRI ROOM

Acoustic noise is generated by the switching of the time-varying gradient magnetic fields.

According to the U.S. Occupational Safety and Health Administration (OSHA) regulations, the Maximum permissible exposure limit (PEL) is 90 dBA for eight hours.

The noise level depends on the strength of the MRI machine, with machines ranging from 0.2 to 3 Tesla producing noise levels from 101 to 131 dB.

Modern 3T MRI scanners are capable of exceeding the PEL and can result in auditory damage to the extent of hearing loss.

While a lesser-known hazard, an increasing number of case reports found evidence of hearing loss following MRI scans.

Texas 2013: The Case of Tinnitus From Lower Back MRI

In 2013 a Texas woman returned with a swollen ear and tinnitus post her lower back MRI scan. She has ever since been living with the constant sounds and opened up about the importance of precautions for MRI auditory damage.

Who are the Potential Risk Bearers for Auditory Damage?

While this can affect anybody undergoing a scan, some patients need special attention :

- All patients undergoing MRI scans especially ones with compromised hearing
- Patient attendants with compromised auditory functions who are inside the MRI Gantry Room during a scan.
- Technical Staff continuously exposed to the MRI Scans and very close to the MRI Bore for longer durations.

THE GOOD NEWS: 11% of Auditory Accidents Can be Avoided by Following These Three Simple Steps.

Just like Burn hazards, preventing Auditory Damage is the easiest to implement.

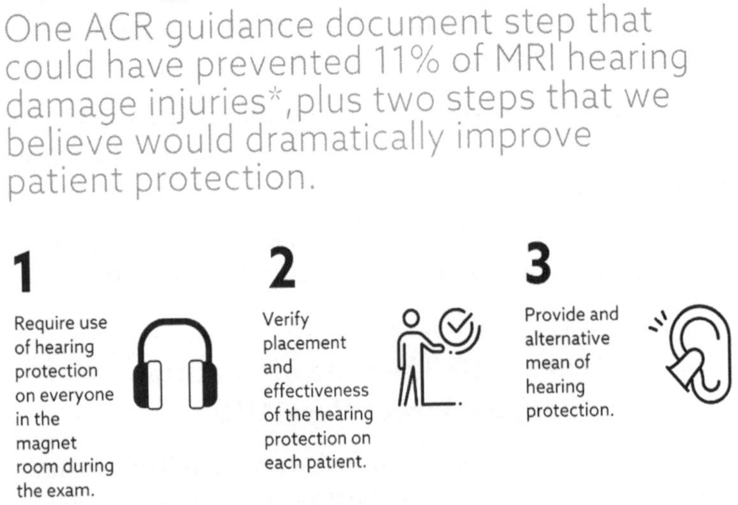
One ACR guidance document step that could have prevented 11% of MRI hearing damage injuries*,plus two steps that we believe would dramatically improve patient protection.
1
Require use of hearing protection on everyone in the magnet room during the exam.
2
Verify placement and effectiveness of the hearing protection on each patient.
3
Provide and alternative mean of hearing protection.

Image Courtesy: Metrasens, UK.

1. Patients should always use MRI Headphones provided by the MRI vendor for all scans.
2. In the case of the use of head coils, if the headphones do not fit, silicon earplugs can be used.
3. There should be hearing protection for attendants (if any) who accompany the patient inside the MRI Gantry.

Shveta's Pro Safety Tip

The screening checklist should have a clear requirement to mention if the patient has an compromised hearing or has recently undergone any treatment for the ear.

Always test the efficacy of the hearing protection aid by calling out to the patient post providing the hearing protection. If they can still hear you, the hearing protection aid is not correctly placed and may need to be changed or readjusted accordingly.

SECRET - 7

THE MASTER SECRET REVEALED THE 3P FRAMEWORK SOLUTION

As per the ACR guidelines 2024: Root cause analyses of MR safety accidents reveal that accidents resulted only very rarely from a malfunction of the MR equipment. Instead, accidents are more typically the result of how the equipment was being used, frequently involving a breakdown in adherence to policies and procedures or being impacted by previously unrecognized significant gaps in those policies and procedures. As there will always be potential for human error, it is essential that MR facilities design thoughtful policies and procedures that reliably address predictable as well as unusual situations.

A few equipment providers are working on analysing the MRI Safety issues and working on solutions to help make MRI Rooms safer. One such company in the UK, Metrasens did a study of MRI accident cases. As per a study done by Metrasens:

- Approximately 95% of all accidents are caused by Ferromagnetic Projectiles, Burns, and Auditory Damage.
- Also, a whopping 74% of these accidents are avoidable, which is a good number to work with.

➢ Developing a foundational framework to prevent these types of accidents would significantly enhance the safety of our MRI environment.

Metrasens analyzed all of the MRI injury accidents reported to the FDA via their MedWatch program in 2015 and 2016 and tested which preventions would be most effective in keeping patients and staff safe.

In total, we reviewed 112 MRI-related injuries. 106 of these were categorized as burns, hearing damage, or injuries caused by projectiles. We looked closer at each of these incidents and evaluated whether best practice recommendations - taken from the ACR Guidance Document on MR Safe Practices (2013)* - could have helped prevent them. We've summarized our analysis below

95%

of reported injuries we analyzed were related to burns, projectiles, or hearing damage.

74%

of these incidents could have been prevented by followint the nine best practices detailed below.

*Image Courtsey: Metrasens, UK.

During my meetings and training programs at various hospitals across India, I have had the opportunity to discuss various accidents that occurred in these facilities. Upon reviewing and analysing the causes of various reported and unreported incidents in Indian hospitals, I identified that there were several factors contributing to these accidents.

All the reasons could be broadly categorised into three heads:

1. Lack of knowledge by the users on the potential hazards. There was also a lack of knowledge about what to do and what not to do to avoid accidents.
2. Lack of the correct devices/equipment/furniture that are safe to be used in the MRI environment. Lack of awareness of the availability of these devices in the market.
3. Lack of awareness or implementation of correct procedures which need to be followed in case any accident happens.

That led me to think if we could develop a framework of implementable points which could be followed so that we can develop a means to avoid the reasons for the above accidents.

That's how I developed -

"Shveta's 3P Framework for Safer MRI Rooms".

The 3P Framework is a simple yet comprehensive and implementable structure through which we identify what could be the potential cause for the accidents and also the areas we need to focus on to ensure we can avoid MRI Accidents.

This framework acts as a guideline for the institutes and helps them figure out where to begin in their quest for safer MRI rooms.

Shveta's 3P Framework for Safer MRI Rooms

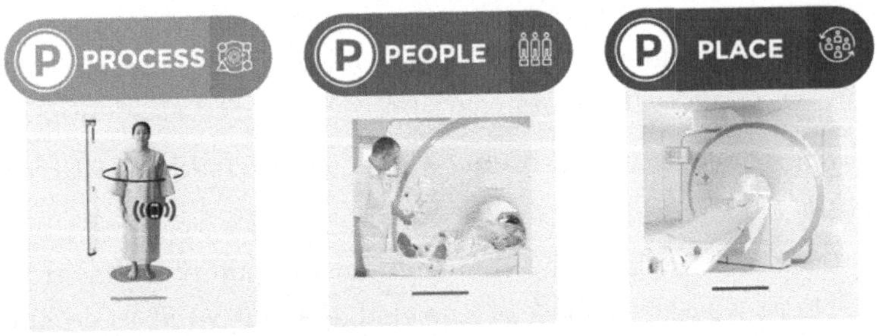

The 3P framework divides the MRI Safety tasks into three heads: Process, People, and Place. Implementing strategies in all these areas can help mitigate multiple MRI safety concerns.

Let's look at each segment of the 3P framework and understand how to implement this in our setup.

1. PROCESS

All hospitals have defined processes for every department that enables people to know what needs to be done and how it needs to be done. While MRI rooms require a separate setup and have a special force in play here , unfortunately, processes are not defined separately for the MRI Environment.

The MRI must have processes that need to be discussed, documented, and thoroughly followed during normal times. A separate set of processes should be made to address the times of emergencies. For example: We need to have documented processes around MRI safety concerns like patient screening processes and processes to be followed in case of an MRI emergency or MRI accident of any kind. These need to be comprehensive, relevant to your facility, and concise. Once these are defined it becomes clear to everyone who has access to the MRI facility on what to do and what not to do in the MRI facility.

The other advantage of documented processes is that in case of an MRI Accident, everyone knows how to proceed and we do not lose any precious time to respond.

SHVETA'S PRO SAFETY TIP

These processes should also be placed in a location where they can be seen by anyone who accesses the MRI.

Including these processes in the onboarding training can also help impart the relevant education to the new joinees who are not fully aware of the MRI Hazards.

2. PEOPLE

People are the backbone of any process. To implement any safety process people need to be well-trained so that they understand the gravity of the above concerns and the need to follow best practices at all times in MRI areas. Anyone who has access to an MRI facility needs to be trained in MRI Safety. These trainings need to be for all disciplines especially focusing on non-radiology departments who end up being in the MRI facility.

These trainings also need to happen on a regular basis so that best practices become a habit. The training can be categorised into two levels.

- **Level 1 MR Personnel:** Level 1 MR Personnel are those who have been educated and successfully mastered MR safety topics as defined by the facility's MRMD to ensure that they would not constitute a danger to themselves or others in the MR environment
- **Level 2 MR Personnel:** Level 2 MR Personnel are those who have been more extensively trained and educated in MR safety topics beyond Level 1 MR training. Due to their higher level of MR safety training and associated job responsibilities, Level 2 MR Personnel supervise Level 1 MR Personnel in MR safety-related aspects of practice.

In addition, all MRIs need to have a dedicated MRI Safety officer identified for their facility.

Shveta's Pro Safety Tip

There should be at least two designated MRI Safety Officers so that we can cover all times including non-working hours.

A special session on MRI Safety should also be organised for the GDA staff who access the area for cleaning purposes.

3. PLACE

The MRI facility needs to be designed to make it safer. It needs to be divided into Zones and segregated clearly as Zones 1,2,3 and 4 as defined in the ACR guidelines. These areas should be monitored and access to the area is to be given to people who are trained and understand the risks involved.

There should be methods and tools to ensure restricted access of devices and people to higher magnetic field areas. Another activity that would be of help is a risk assessment of your facility by an independent body at least once a year to be able to identify the hazards and mitigate the risks.

The MRI environment is different from the other hospital areas and requires products that are tested to work in the high magnetic fields of the MRI. There are so many products available today that can help make your MRI facility safer and easier to use.

There is a lack of knowledge and clarity on how to identify this equipment. The teams should ensure that the MRI Zones only have the equipment that is conditional and approved to be used in those Zones. Also, any equipment in Zone 3 and Zone 4 should be clearly identified and labelled as per the MRI guidelines and used accordingly. Appropriate training can help in identifying these products and reading the labels.

Another key aspect here is to ensure no non-conditional equipment accidentally enters the MRI facility which can help avoid many projectile accidents.

Working on the above Process, People and Place sections is a great start.

However, it is important to note that each MRI facility is

different and a one-shoe-fits-all approach might not be the ideal one. This is the onus of the radiology department to use these as guidelines to begin their MRI safety journey. Customising the solution basis your facility yet adhering to the basic guidelines is the key here. In case of doubts, there are individual consultants available who can analyse the facility and highlight the requirements and help implement the safety measures here.

In case you are still unsure about how to begin, we have documented the first and simplest steps for you.

Read on to know more...

SECRET - 8

THE WAY FORWARD

While MRI Safety in itself requires a deep study and analysis for implementation there is a start strategy that we could recommend that will help you begin your MRI Safety journey.

As mentioned previously, any recommendations need to be weighed in light of your department's workflow and the best solution adapted accordingly.

So if you are ready to begin this journey let me share the first steps.

Your department could begin with the below three areas basis the 3P framework.

PROCESS: Comprehensive and Documented

The right processes can help prevent accidents and provide clear guidelines for actions to be taken. The key decision-makers and stakeholders should collectively work on these process lists. Involving other disciplines who regularly use the MRI facility would also be a good idea.

- Prepare patient screening documented checklist – comprehensive but concise and as applicable to your hospital. This checklist should fit well in your workflow.

- Prepare a checklist for the radiology staff which they can refer to on a daily basis to follow.
- Define a checklist for non-radiology staff to ensure they are safe before they enter the MRI Zones.
- Policies and Procedures to be defined for how to handle emergencies like cardiac arrest, and quench. These documents should clearly define the steps to be followed to avoid losing precious time during an emergency
- Policies and procedures documents should be placed in a location that is accessible by all working in the MRI room.
- Identify and designate an MRI Safety Officer for your facility.

PEOPLE: Trained and Aware

- For the right processes to be implemented in the right way people need to be made aware of the importance of MRI Safety. Conduct MRI safety training for staff of all disciplines at regular intervals. The MRI trainings should cover the basics of MRI Hazards and practical implementation on how to avoid them.
- Define an MRI training Calendar to ensure this activity is done regularly and religiously
- Include MRI Safety training in the Hospital Onboarding checklist.
- Identify one resource as an MRI Safety Officer who along with ensuring department safety is also responsible for overseeing the pieces of training.

Sample Training Framework for MRI Safety Training

Radiologists / MRI Technicians Once in 6 months

- Types of MRI damages
- Common Causes
- Mitigation methods
- Patient Safety for implants, contrasts, pregnancy
- Resources available
- Certification course

Anaesthesiologists Once in 6 months

- Why MRI safety is important
- How MRI Environment
- is different from normal ICU/OT: MHD effect
- Equipment available for patient safety in MRI
- Emergency Checklist

Hospital Staff Once in a quarter

- Why MRI is different?
- What is MRI Safety ?
- What to do and not do when approaching an MRI Room

PLACE: Analysed and Access Control Zoned

This should be your first step and you could start immediately.

➢ Analyse your department and identify different Zones and how you can ensure restricted access to the magnetic field area

➢ Identify the required MRI conditional equipment – monitors, wheelchairs, syringe pumps, and stethoscopes- and label them the same.

➢ Do a thorough risk assessment of your facility and identify the evident hazards.

➢ Develop a risk mitigation plan using the concepts above.

Another key here is to ensure MRI equipment is stored and used exclusively in the MRI facility and there is less interexchange of these with other department equipment.

USA: The Case of The Suspicious Nose Magnets in Colorado

During a patient screening at the Children's Hospital of Colorado, a potential patient injury-causing ferrous object was found. A 14-year-old needed an abdominal MRI. After the patient completed the standard screening form and verbal evaluation the patient seemed safe to be scanned. The hospital uses a ferromagnetic screener for implant detection. The FMDS scanning led to alertness for ferromagnetic objects present on the patient.

The staff refused to scan till a complete investigation was done on the alarm. Subsequent X-ray showed small magnets on the nasal septum thereby saving an MRI accident.

The incident not only reveals the hospital's commitment to MRI safety and using ferromagnetic detection systems, but it is also a great example of how combining a place using correct MRI products, having the right processes, and people trained to understand the alerts and triggers helped prevent a potential accident.

Also, this example clearly shows that if you follow the basics of MRI Safety protocols it can help you achieve:

- MRI Safe environments for your patients and your teams.
- Loss of hospital reputation can be avoided.
- Financial benefits from MRI Safe rooms.

HOW CAN WE HELP?

The 3P model developed by Shveta Dang is a great place to start and can be followed to achieve most of your desired results.

An understanding and acceptance of unique requirements for MRI is the key. MRI SAFETY is achievable if we focus on the same.

To recap what we have learned :

- Focus on training people to understand how the MRI room is different and how important it is to focus on MRI Safety.
- Focus on process-driven workflow. Every interaction in the MRI environment needs to be thought about carefully and efficient processes formulated to help keep the MRI safe.
- Focus on Place to ensure you only have certified MRI conditional equipment both in Zone 4 and Zone 3.

The concepts mentioned above are a great start to your MRI journey. However, given the huge load on the medical ecosystem in India, you might have issues specific to your site. We do understand that your site might need more attention and a customised solution

Also please note that A BOOK DOES HAVE PAGE CONSTRAINTS which do not allow us to detail all the points mentioned.

As an MRI Safety Enthusiast, I am happy to offer my help at any time.

In case you need more details or want in-depth information analysis, I invite you to reach out to us to be able to schedule a full session on any of the below:

- Discussion on online/offline training of your teams.
- Discussion regarding doing a site audit for your site and submitting a report with our analysis.
- Help you build a checklist for your department.

- Understand the current functioning both from Radiology and other stakeholder perspectives and Assess the current risk areas.
- Recommend mitigation plans basis the 3P approach, especially for place and process.
- Work with the departments to implement your MRI Safety plans.
- In case of a new MRI coming up, provide valuable inputs for the zoning of your facility.

To begin our journey together I invite you to enroll in the MRI Safety In India Community.

For the readers of this book, the subscription is FREE!

- Once you enroll you will also get FREE access to
- Patient Scanning Form
- Sample Safety Checklists can be a starting point for you and can be customised for your facilities.

This will give you access to connect with other like-minded community members. Also, I will be regularly updating the community with information from my series:

Mastering MRI Safety: Stay Safe, Scan Smart.

Once you enroll you will also get FREE access to Patient Sample Safety Checklists that can be a starting point for you and can be customised for your facilities.

Scan the QR Code to enroll now.

In case you need any help you could drop an email to: **shveta@marrsis-disha.com** or schedule a call with me on **+91 9958111400.**

MRI Safety begins with you, me, and everyone. It's important for us to understand the risks involved and educate the stakeholders about the same.

We as an organization are dedicating our time to promoting MRI safety and I do believe we can achieve safer and accident-free MRIs soon.

Until then, wish you luck in your MRI Safety Journey.

BIBLIOGRAPHY

- ACR Guidelines Manual 2024
- Metrasens, UK website
- Gilk Radiology Consultant.com
- https://www.dnaindia.com/mumbai/report-mumbai-mri-death-case-freak-mishap-turns-into blame-game-2579317
- https://www.hindustantimes.com/india-news/uttar-pradesh-minister-s-guard-carries-gun-during-mri-scan-ruins-machine/story-H3hOPJMU5xpXoTtI6bBBaO.html
- Metrasens, UK resources
- https://pubs.rsna.org/doi/abs/10.1148/rg.230102?journalCode=radiographics
- https://www.telegraph.co.uk/news/uknews/1458421/Pacemaker-death-after-error-in-hospital.html
- https://x.com/tobiasgilk/status/1590343462536155136?mx=2
- https://www.mid-day.com/mumbai/mumbai-news/article/mumbai-man-sucked-in-by-mri-machine-gets-away-with-just-a-broken-finger-23183247